Differently Human

Emma Leigh

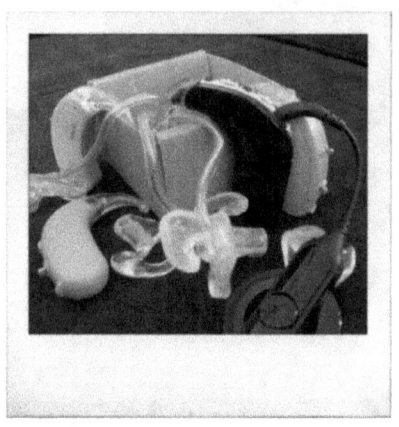

Opening Pandora's Box

Emma Leigh asserts the moral right to be identified as the author of this work.

Cover Photograph © Glen Leigh

Going...

Losing your hearing in your early twenties is fortunately a rare occurrence – however, it happened to me. Sometimes I think that I must have been deaf before that and never noticed – but that simply wasn't the case – I once was a hearing person, but now am not.

In the UK, around one person in seven is deaf or hard of hearing.

The most common cause of hearing loss is ageing. Three-quarters of people who are deaf are aged over 60. According to the charity, Deafness Research UK, age-related hearing loss normally begins at around 50. But it's not just older people who are affected.

Being exposed to too much loud noise is an important cause of hearing loss. It is thought that loud noise is behind the increasing numbers of young people who are losing their hearing. The popularity of MP3 players and other personal music systems, and pubs and clubs that play very loud music, all contribute.

The one that is not often mentioned is the link to underlying medical conditions – or just plain bad luck- as is the case with me.

...Going...

Most of us take our hearing for granted, so it's easy not to notice at first when it goes.

It's usually a gradual process. Background noises start to sound a little blurry, you can't make out quiet voices and you don't hear announcements at airports and train stations.

Next, you have difficulties hearing what people are saying if there's background chatter, especially if it's a child speaking or someone who's quietly spoken.

Then you find that in a busy setting you have to concentrate really hard on what the person you're talking to is saying and you start to pay more attention to people's lip movements and expressions to read what you can't hear.

Gone?

This book tells the story of my cochlear implant operation – the before (my thoughts as the operation date drew closer), the middle (the operation and recovery) and the after (waiting for the big switch on). Writing things down was an important process for me – but I also come to hope that my story would be useful to someone else in the future; after all there is little literature available for young adults who become deafened.

At the back of the book you will find some general information about the implant process – whilst it is not intended to provide a definitive guide hopefully it will fill in a few gaps about what is a complicated process.

And so the countdown to my "cochlear implantation" begins...

So today, with just 16 sleeps to go, I'm going to start letting you into my inner ramblings on my journey towards Cochlear Implantation.

For those who don't know me - "Hello I'm Emma!" - thanks for joining me on what I expect to be the roller coaster ride to end all roller coaster rides.

So yes, here I am - 37 years young (wife, mum of two, full-time employee and some time Masters student) - no hearing left, hoping to make the best of a not-so-great situation.

A bit of background... where I was just three years ago

I wasn't born deaf; I started to lose my hearing in my very early twenties. At that point I had been married to my hubby for 5 years and had two children (yeah I am an early starter!).

I currently have two degrees *show-off alert* one of them being a Creative Writing Degree. For one of my assignments I was asked to do a piece of life writing, on a subject which changed the direction of my life - so here's a snippet!

Life, part two

Sometimes the changes which happen in life are so subtle that they blend into one another so smoothly, seamlessly. With the relentless hustle and bustle of bringing up a young family the last thing I wanted to acknowledge was the fact that I was losing my precious hearing; I was born into a hearing world and wanted to remain there. I loved to talk and to listen to other people; I didn't want anything to alter that. So as defiant and stubborn as ever I made it my business to ignore the fact, refusing to acknowledge that a cataclysmic change was happening in my life whether I liked it or not. Fast forwards a couple of years and here I am with only 5% of my residual hearing left, which to those not familiar with 'hearing impaired' terminology means I am profoundly deaf. Even with the assistance of my digital hearing aids I am only able to achieve approximately 60% of what I might be able to hear – that's 6 out of every 10 words spoken, try and imagine constantly trying to fill in the gaps.

Just for a moment let me rewind back to the beginning. At the early stages of my hearing loss it was very easy to continue life in a normal fashion, turning up the volume of the TV a fraction is not a massive upheaval in the wider scheme of life. Turning myself into a dizzy social butterfly, asking people to repeat themselves when snatches of conversation were a jumble was a harder task; hoping that my newly acquired acting skills distracted them from my hearing problems – after all, being deaf was something I thought happened to older people as a natural progression, not to young adults like me. Little did I realise at this time was that the grieving process had already begun and that I was at the very cusp of mourning the person that I no longer was or was ever going to become.

Children have a bizarrely accurate way of summing up a situation which adults often find challenging to articulate. I can vividly recall a conversation which I had with my then 5 year old daughter. It was on one of those days when things seem to be almost perfect, with all the clichés intact. The sky was cloudless and an amazing shade of blue, the surrounding countryside was beginning to flush out the weariness of winter with a spray paint of dazzling green. I was driving my little one home from school, chattering away about the day when I happened to mention that mummy was thinking of getting some hearing aids to help make her hear better. Almost immediately the atmosphere changed from being bright and sunny to ominously dark and foreboding. "I don't want a mummy who wears black corks in her ears," said my sweet little girl with a frown on her face. I can remember feeling as though I had been physically kicked in my stomach as we continued the journey home in silence, my head spinning with the thought that my child wanted a normal mummy, not one with an impairment.

No matter what changes are taking place in our lives the days, weeks and months continue to pass whether we like it or not. Unfortunately for me my hearing loss reached the point where I could no longer pretend that it wasn't affecting my life and my tentative steps into the 'deaf' world began. Something needed to be done. Looking back now it seems quite clear that an element of acceptance about my new situation was entering my consciousness, though at the time I can recall feeling like a reluctant toddler who wanted to stamp their feet in utter frustration. Endless hearing tests became an enduring feature of my life together with the frequent trips to the local audiology department with its posters advertising sign language classes and deaf clubs, which make me laugh for all the wrong reasons as you never see 'hearing clubs' advertised! To this day I have an incredibly bittersweet relationship with the audiology department. Part of me is totally humbled with gratitude that such places exist and that I am provided with hearing aids which give me some semblance of a life. The other part of me hates and despises the place as my visits, even years later, frustrate and depress me due to the fact that I know the staff will never be able to provide me the ultimate cure, a pair of fully functioning ears.

And so my diary begins and life, part three

Becoming Differently Human

A troubled day

I don't think I ever fully appreciated that I would ever get to this chapter, the third period of re-invention and trying to define or even find out who I am.

Of course I was always told that my deafness was progressive, but now I'm actually at the stage of 'implantation' I've suddenly found myself in a blur of uncertainty.

Yes, **implantation,** what a word – it sounds like a foreign body being inserted against a person's will – which, in a way, I suppose that's what it is – except of course I've agreed that's what I want.

Some stuff – the cochlear implant should be a good thing, it is... I'll look back at these ramblings and laugh, hopefully.

Let me try and justify today's thought processes... I'm feeling sad because I hate that something is going to happen to me that I've always wanted to avoid, yet welcome it at the same time... weird.

I'm feeling sad because I should be feeling happy that I have got this opportunity to try and make the best of a bad situation – AKA – being profoundly deaf.

I'm feeling frustrated because I can't do the simplest thing – actually tell the people around me about what's going to happen.

So let's investigate this a bit further.

Reasons why I can't actually tell people:

The words get stuck in my throat, ha ha (yes really!!)

I feel like I am making myself look deficient in some way

I don't want to see expressions of sympathy or pity – I'm not dead after all!

Any great insights there? I'll let you be the psychologist today.

Another day closer...

Number of sleeps remaining until implantation: 14

Today's thoughts: Outside the bubble

Another busy day to take my mind off thinking about what's coming up in the next two weeks (that's two weeks TODAY)

Even IKEA played a role in distraction techniques today - LOL - the powers of Swedish meatballs :)

A big day tomorrow - I'm going to hospital for the final appointment before doomsday. Another battery of hearing tests (on the off chance that a miracle has happened and I've regained my hearing) and I get to select my 'device'.

An interesting concept really - choosing what gets embedded in your skull.

A day of two halves (or maybe three thirds...)

Number of sleeps remaining until implantation: 13

Today's thoughts: Who am I?

A day of two halves really...

Last night, despite my attempts to wear myself out by walking the whole IKEA circuit, found me tossing and turning at 1am.

Consequently it didn't put me in the best frame of mind for today's visit.

Today - Part 1

I was presented with a 'colleague recognition award' at work, after 7 - yes you read that correctly 7 people nominated me! I must admit it felt a little weird having all those nice things read out about me - it felt like they were being said about someone else.

What started out as a happy occasion ultimately made me feel sad - will I ever achieve anything like that again??

Today - Part 2

Fortunately the trip to hospital was wrapped up in just 2.5 hours today.

First I 'tried on' various sound processors, in order to pick my future ear companion. Mmmm it was a tricky decision, but in the end I chose a... (You'll have to wait and see!)

I then met my surgeons and was read the riot act about things which could go wrong...

A trip to get vaccinated against meningitis

Finally an epic pre-op session with the friendliest nurse you'll ever meet.

AND THAT'S IT - I've signed on the dotted line.

Right now... I could easily kick back and enjoy a glass of wine, but study calls.

Calm... (I think!)

Number of sleeps remaining until implantation: 12

Today's thought: Tales of the unexpected

Hello readers, thanks for sticking with me.

Oddly I feel rather calm today, perhaps too calm...

I'm beginning to wonder if the meningitis injection was actually some kind of sedative.

Well at least I'm not having a high, low, high, low day.

I guess today's big announcement, was my err.... smallish announcement in my team meeting at work - explaining briefly about my forthcoming December absence.

A few surprised faces, and a lot of kind words - I was incredibly touched.

Received the official inpatient letter today - I need to arrive at the hospital by 4pm on the 5th of December (wonder if I will get a 'light' Welsh tea???).

The op is then scheduled for 9am on the Monday morning - which will last for at least 3 hours. I'm actually looking forward to the uninterrupted sleep :)

A proper weird day all round

Number of sleeps remaining until implantation: 11

Today's thoughts: Letting go...

Gosh - Thursday already! Where has the week gone? I know I wanted to keep myself distracted but...

Well how's today been, bit on the weird side really - which seems to have been the popular consensus. (Glad I'm not alone in my weirdness)

Thinking about letting go, of the person who I think I am now, the person I was never going to be - will the real 'Emma' please step forwards?

Losing my hearing sparked a kind of grieving process - and it took time. My memories of being a hearing person are still very vivid even now. Even though I can't hear the sounds I can still 'hear' the sounds in my head (gosh I'm making myself upset here, but hey, better out than in)

Things I can remember clearly:

- Taking my French Oral Exam at school, I could actually hear and speak in French!

- My Nanna's voice - it was pretty 'unique'

- My wedding day, saying my vows, repeating what the registrar said word perfect.

- My first baby crying, mewling away. Weirdly (sorry - it's word of the day) I could even hear her crying from the hospital nursery where she had been taken so I could get some sleep. I instinctively knew it was my baby.

What I can hear now (without the hearing aids that is!):

- Occasionally, low sounding rumbles...

- Most of the time, nowt at all

But being deaf is not a quiet experience - tinnitus rings away, or sometimes twitters away like an odd morning chorus - yep you've guessed it - weird!

And another thing

Number of sleeps remaining until implantation: still 11

"Wanting to be someone else is a waste of the person you are."

~ Kurt Cobain

Well that's me told...

Friday, Friday

Number of sleeps remaining until implantation: 10

Today's thoughts: Take a walk in another person's shoes

Today the boot has definitely been on the other foot, so to speak.

I'm so used to being the patient; today it is my turn to be the nurse to my Hubby. Of course, it has been the role in the past but today I've paced around like a mad thing. It got me wondering, do people pace around when they are waiting for me to return from noxious slumber??

Since my patient is resting (sleeping!) I'll try and write of few words about today.

Anyway, back to walking in another person's shoes... Today I had a conversation about appreciating what you have - in other words making the best of things you have. I suppose it ties in with Kurt's words from yesterday.

It's a common truth that there is always someone who is worse off than you - that I DO NOT dispute. But its strange how when we are faced with a challenge, we feel like we are the only person to have ever have faced it (I can just imagine you all saying, for goodness sake - get over yourself will you!)

Anyway, so here is a bit of a dilemma - do we face our challenges with the attitude it's OK (whatever it is) because there is someone worse off than you, or do we allow our self to recognise that we ARE facing a challenge and no matter what, it's OK to have a few wobbles along the way?

For me I guess I need that permission to have a wobble now and again without thinking I'm letting everyone down.

Anxiety hour update

Number of sleeps remaining until implantation: still 10, but it's officially anxiety hour so...

"Genius might be the ability to say a profound thing in a simple way"

~ Charles Bukowski

Not really anything to do with today, by Charles Bukowski is a great author!

An early morning rant...

Number of sleeps remaining until implantation: 9 (gulp - single figures)

Today's thoughts: (*insert ranting words of choice*)

Morning.

Please excuse this early morning rant - but as I want to accurately document my journey - I'm going to have to.

Isn't it amazing how one person's thoughtless/ignorant comments can undo the progress made in a week?

Yesterday, Hubby decided to 'inform' Mother In Law about my impending surgery.

I'll quit waffling - this is the 'highlight'

H: Emma's have the implant surgery done in December.

MIL: She never said...

(Much waffling...)

MIL: Well she does well to do the job she does considering...

H: Considering what???

(I was actually in the room while this conversation was going on)

Yep - it seems we're back to the old "deaf=stupid" scenario. I thought I had done my best to challenge that - hell what should I be 'capable' of doing - sitting in my pyjamas and watching TV all day??????

I'm expecting today to continue on a similar vein as I am going to tell my own mother and brother (Father will have to hear from Mother...).

Stand back all and don your flak jackets and hard helmets.

Today, part deux

Number of sleeps remaining until implantation: 9, if it happens

Today's thoughts: "..... speechless....."

Well, I've calmed down somewhat - and might I add I'm very fond of my MIL - just wish she'd think a little more about what she says.

So... I told my Brother and Mother.

The response...

SILENCE

No matter how old you are it seems you still have the ability to shock your Mother!

Thank goodness for my 8 year old Godson who piped up, "can I send you a card Aunty Emma?" - Bless :)

Anyway, during shopping with Mother, she enquired about my dressing gown and slippers status - it's a start I suppose.

So that's it - most people now know.

My minds a total jumble - just hope I can get through the next week unscathed.

Scary dream visitor

Number of sleeps remaining until implantation: 8 (hopefully with no more Pennywise)

Today's thoughts: News of the World

What a night last night...

Tired after a Christmas shopping marathon I was expecting a rather good night's sleep.

Okay, the stuff with MIL and my own Mother was grating me a bit - but the last thing I expected was a night of dreaming about Pennywise the Clown (From Stephen King's IT, in case you're not familiar).

What on earth is that all about???

Whenever, I closed my eyes to go back to sleep Pennywise would be there again, opening and closing doors to scare me.

Are my worries translating themselves into clowns???

A week of lasts

Number of sleeps remaining until implantation: 7

Today's thoughts: A foot in both worlds, belonging in none

Yep - bit melancholy today.

This time next week the deed will be done - I (or the surgeons) will have obliterated my cochlear, I will never be able to use a hearing aid again - and to top it all I'll have a charming bald patch.

Yeah yeah, the upshot is that I will be a different kind of deaf person.

I think this is what is called a tiny moment of doubt.

So anyway, a foot in both worlds, belonging in none sums up how I am feeling today. Even with the operation it's not really going to change that is it?

Hmmmm.....

Weird dream again last night (yeah I know its b o r i n g listening to other people's dreams...).

In my dream it was Sunday and a nurse was showing me to my bed. However, when we got to what was to be my room it was like a prison door. Inside the room were three beds, covered with black sheets - and I couldn't decide which bed I should get in to.

Hmmmm... it was most strange - going to have to Google a dream dictionary or something.

Uncanny

Number of sleeps remaining until implantation: still 7

Just browsed a dream dictionary - couldn't find anything about black sheets, but found the following about Clowns (not Pennywise specifically but...)

CLOWN: The obvious meaning of clowns is that you feel foolish or that you may have been seen as an object of ridicule who cannot be taken seriously. But clowns also can be linked more frequently to false emotions. They may symbolise someone who is not dealing with some trauma very well - putting on a brave face and not really dealing with emotional upset.

OMG - I'm obvious, even when I'm not being obvious...

Number of sleeps remaining: 6

Today's thoughts until implantation: Friendship

Not so great today, bit of a cold I can't shift and stress headache...

Friendship is my theme of the day, in its many guises. So thanks to those who are there, thanks to those who share happy news, thanks to my Uncle who sent me a really kind email - I'm lucky to be surrounded by you all. I'm a great believer that people come into your life for a reason, a season or a lifetime.

You've got a friend in me

When the road looks rough ahead

And you're miles and miles

From your nice warm bed

Just remember what your old pal said

Boy, you've got a friend in me

You've got a friend in me

You've got troubles; well I've got 'em too

There isn't anything I wouldn't do for you

We stick together and we see it through

You've got a friend in me

"Toy Story"

Number of sleeps remaining until implantation: 5

Today's thoughts: Black

Not a good day, full of black thoughts.

Spent my working today delivering a training session - will I ever do that in the future (well... yes tomorrow as I am also delivering the same session again...) - But you know what I mean?

Tried to think how I would feel if it was Hubby who was having the operation and not me, I've seen the stress that this is causing him - what right do I have to do that to anyone, especially the closest person to me? What about my children?

This whole thing is MASSIVE.

Blackness

Number of sleeps remaining until implantation: 5

Things not what they used to be

Missing one inside of me

Deathly lost, this can't be real

Can't stand this hell I feel

~ Metallica

Fade to Black

(Hoping for a lighter day tomorrow)

Number of sleeps remaining until implantation: 4

Today's thought: Absolutely void

Feel a bit better than I did last night, managed a good night's sleep - which always helps.

Delivered my last training session, as me as I am now - and how do I feel about that, well...see today's 'thoughts'.

My son, seemed to have a bit of a wobble this morning. I can see he is scared for me (and also about who will make tea in my absence!! - he's dreaming of take-outs!!) It's not fair for a 15 year old to have these kinds of worries, the poor kid had seen me treated for cancer and as a parent it's certainly not a memory that you want to create in your child's childhood. It's the same for my daughter, although she has her own life now, she still worries for her Mump.

Had a bit of a strange email from my other Uncle, he did a 'Mother' and never acknowledged the 'news' - so guess it isn't news to him.

No word from my Father...

Thank goodness for my own little family - without them I would be totally alone.

So if there are any families out there looking for information on implants and you happen to be reading this book - the best advice from me, please show some your implantee some support.

Number of sleeps remaining until implantation: 3

Today's thoughts: Is this it?

Well, I've just finished work - the 'out of office' is on, so Emma is officially out of the building.

For now I can't imagine walking back through the door, the familiar suddenly feels very unfamiliar.

Wish I had a time machine so that I could see how things will be this time next week.

I think there is something to be said for 'living for the moment', so why on earth I am trying to live in the future?

Thanks to those who have been there today, your kindness and friendship has meant a great deal.

Number of sleeps remaining until implantation: 2

Today's thoughts: Bit too early for thoughts yet...

Well, it's 6.24am and I've been awake for the last hour or so.

So far I've got one load of washing done and have watched an episode of Neighbours on Sky+.

It feels a bit like the day before Christmas Eve, you know, when you still have loads to do.

So today's task list!

- Food shop for the next two weeks (Hubby has kindly offered to put the Christmas tree up while my son and I do this)

- Buy new slippers and cosy PJ's (you can never have too many pairs of slippers)

- Make 'early Christmas dinner' (My daughter and BF are coming to visit, soooo excited)

- Sort pets out

- Sort out bag for hospital

- Google cochlear implants some more just in case there is anything I've missed

- Ummmm... panic some more

Number of sleeps remaining until implantation: 1

Today's thought: IT'S here (see earlier entry for a link to 'IT')

Well, it's 7.49am and I've actually managed to have quite a decent sleep.

Had a great day yesterday with the early Christmas activity, the meal was delicious - even though I say so myself :)

I need to be at the hospital for 4pm, or maybe 2pm - depending on which letter I read (so I am going to go with the middle-man and aim for 3pm) - goodness knows why I need to be there quite that early. Perhaps I've got a final round of hearing tests to look forward to. I am wondering at which point they can going to shave my hair off...

Let battle commence.

Number of sleeps remaining until implantation: 1

15 hours to go

Well, I'm now here at Glan Clwyd.

It took me less than 15 minutes to become an impatient patient, though the staff seem very kind and don't mind me mithering on about my hair.

I am in a side room of my own, with a TV which has subtitles (!!), my own 'facilities' and a really odd bed with numerous controls.

I've just had my tea, soup (think it might have been chicken), quiche and trifle. I was rather hungry and wolfed it down, possibly a little too quickly.

So far it feels very weird, I'm in hospital yet not ill!

Number of sleeps remaining until implantation: A couple of hours if I'm lucky

10 hours to go...

So I'm now 'nil by mouth', don't think I could stomach anything anyway.

I can honestly say these last few weeks have felt like living hell - I hope dear reader that you never have to make this kind of decision.

When Hubby left the hospital, he said 'goodbye' to my left ear (or my left hearing aid) - that started the tears, just when you thought you are all cried out, there are always a few more waiting. However, he was right, my trusty left hearing aid has served me well - it has let me feel like part of the hearing world.

Oh, and another thing - my hair is being shaved off in the morning.

Number of sleeps remaining until implantation: 0

Today's thoughts: See you on the other side

It's 7.38am; I'm already missing a significant chunk of hair. I always wondered what I would look like with a skinhead, now I know.

I'm prepped for theatre, so just sat here waiting for it all to happen now.

What I am thinking/feeling? Dunno really, feel a bit sickly, but on the whole I just want it over, and of course I am going to get my wish now. (Thank goodness I hear you collectively say!)

I'll write some more when I can - but a sincere thanks to all for putting up with me over the last month or so - I know I have been difficult to be around. I hope that in the future there will be some small way that I can repay your kindness.

Now tomorrow's here today

And yesterday's today's just fade away

~ Perfect

Lightning Seeds

Going, going, gone

I guess it would be handy to show you the stages of 'preparation'

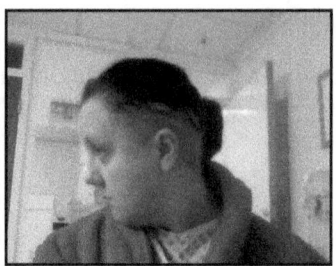

This is the first attempt at prepping me for theatre… before the nurse decided she needed another attempt…

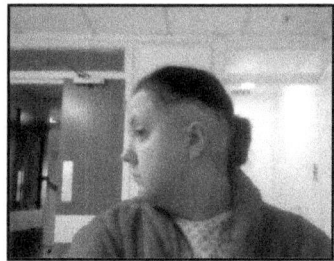

As you can see by this point the nurse had been creative with her razor skills.

And finally… the following morning – they certainly don't scrimp on bandages.

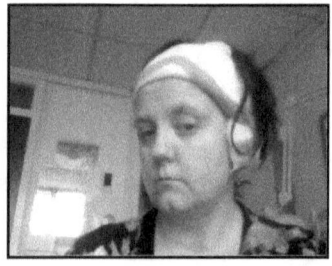

Number of sleeps since implantation: 1

Today's thought: Dizzy

Well I'm still here, which is always a good sign.

Because my heads still a bit whizzy, I'll try and do a list of what happened yesterday (well what I can remember anyway!)

7am - hair shaved off, prepped for theatre.

7.30am - more hair shaved off... not happy bunny at that point.

8.45am - taken to theatre, all useful veins disappeared, cue lots of good natured arm slapping.

9.20am - went to sleeeeeeep

2.30pm - think I can recall being brought back from theatre. Lots of bleeding from head area.

4pm - nurse asked me if I was hungry - world first - Emma said no!

5-7pm - seemed to be given lots of injections, started my vomit marathon...

7pm - Hubby arrived, with cute new bear.

8-9pm - continuation of vomit marathon, more injections and put on a drip

11pm - woke up to find my hand had swelled to enormous proportions (weird...)

5am - woke up again to drip inserted in other hand - suddenly felt v. hungry so had coffee and biscuits.

And now, the doctors have been to visit and have told me I'm to go for an x-ray to check everything is where it should be (might ask them to have a look at my hand too).

If I behave and be a good patient, they will let me go home tomorrow.

So that's it really. If yesterday was the worse I am going to feel, then thank goodness it's over and done with.

Number of sleeps since implantation: 2

Today's thought: Pixie Ear

Today's big news is the removal of the bandages to reveal my new head artwork.

To be fair, the surgeons have done a great job, very neat and tidy - though I do feel a bit like Ms. Frankenstein.

Weirdly, I seem have had some sort of 'ear job' at the same time and I am now supporting a left pixie style ear (which I'm pretty certain I never had to start with).

I am now home from hospital, a touch woozy, but all in one piece. I have been sent home with a plethora of medications, which I DO need to take as the operation site and my neck are quite painful.

I must admit I am finding it very difficult to sit still though; I am such a bad patient.

Tomorrow I'm hoping to get my hair sorted out, though goodness knows what the hairdresser will suggest, other than a full skin head. However, I do like today's style - a side ponytail and scarf!

I think I might need a nap now.

In case you are a little squeamish... look away now!

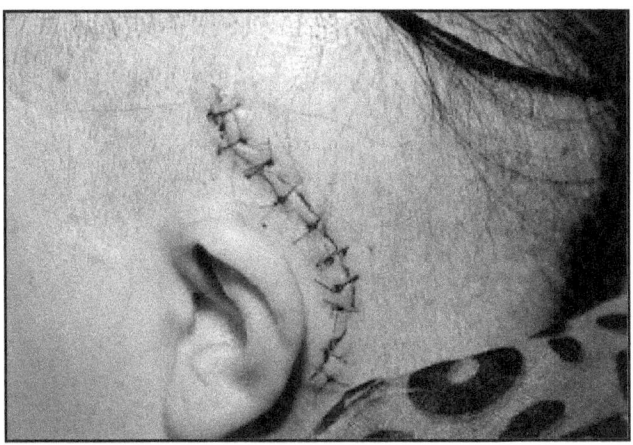

Photo thanks to © Glen Leigh

As you can probably tell me ear does indeed look a little pixie(ish) – possibly due to the tightness of the stitches.

Number of sleeps since implantation: 3

Today's thoughts: Gobbledygook

Gosh my head is spinning, can't see in straight lines at the moment, so hopefully the spellchecker will keep this entry in line.

The dizziness feels like being drunk, without the drink - the thought of alcohol is enough to turn my stomach...

Have tried to do some practical stuff today - had to sort out my sick note after forgetting to ask for one in Wales, the poor locum doctor had a shock when I removed my headscarf.

Other than that, I've had my hair cut, by a hairdresser this time. Sharon has done a great job, I'm impressed.

Need my afternoon sleep now.

Number of sleeps since implantation: 4

Today's thoughts: When will everything stop spinning?

Gosh - what a week.

Can't believe it's only a week since I finished work (LOL what did I used to do???), so much seems to have happened.

I'm in quite a bit of pain at the moment, it feels like someone has stuck a knitting needle in my ear and is poking my brain... sorry, that's a bit graphic - but it blinking well hurts.

The stitches are tight too, so painkillers every 4 hours are the much needed order of the day.

Have started trying to think what it might be that I want from life, part three (when the painkillers have taken effect and the room has stopped spinning, that is!)

So far, I have put my Uni studies on hold (what on earth I was trying to prove to myself I'll never know). I have decided to re-start them again in May 2011 - but am going to go back to studying Psychology.

Ummm... and that's it for today really.

Number of sleeps since implantation: 5

Today's thoughts: A mini meltdown

I'm bawling my eyes out here...

I'm in pain and for the first time I'm wondering what I have let myself in for - I think the euphoria of the operation has well and truly worn off.

Just read this on another CI site:

"When you become a cyborg, you're no less human than you were before" ~ Michael Chorost

---

The essence of 'being human' is something which really bothers me.

> "We do not believe in ourselves until someone reveals that deep inside us is something valuable, worth listening to, worthy of our trust, sacred to our touch. Once we believe in ourselves, we can risk curiosity, wonder, spontaneous delight or any experience that reveals the human spirit"
>
> ~ e.e. Cummings

Number of sleeps since implantation: 6

Today's thoughts: Is my head magnetic?

Feeling roughly the same today. Yesterday Hubby and I ventured out to visit a garden centre to stave off cabin fever.

It was an odd experience as I kept having to turn in full circles in order to work out which direction sound was coming from - which in turn made me even more dizzy.

It was good to get out further than the backyard, but it has taken the wind out of my sails today, so I have had several naps.

My stitches are very irritating, so can't wait for Tuesday to get them removed - just hoping that my head doesn't pop apart...

Number of sleeps since implantation: 7

Today's thoughts: Re: Yesterday's thoughts - no it's not...

Today Hubby and I went to Chester, to finalise the Christmas shopping and to have a bit of time out.

We are making a right pair, Hubby with his knee, me with my zip head. Well, as you can imagine, it was a touch slow going. Fortunately it wasn't too busy (since everyone must be pretty spent up by now) so we ambled along, which turned into me walking too fast, then wondering where Hubby was as I couldn't hear him (cue lots of full body spins to find him).

We had lunch out (ha ha, BOGOF Turkey dinner!!!) and then coffee and cake (and shared painkillers in the afternoon).

Boy does my head hurt now, so I'm trying to drag the time out until painkiller time, so that I can get a semi-decent sleep - have fallen into a habit of waking up at 3.30am for more sminks (AKA 'big pink painkillers').

Off to Glan Clwyd again tomorrow to get the stitches removed and to start using the scar reduction stuff (bless - the hospital noticed I have a slightly unsightly scar on my neck thanks to thyroid cancer, they thought they would provide some extra help this time round - except my hair will cover it...). I'm also hoping that I get my activation date and rehab appointments sorted out too, am starting to feel the need for some structure and forward planning.

Number of sleeps since implantation: 8

**Today's thoughts: Re: Re: Yesterdays and the day before -
actually it is**

Today was 'stitches out' day at Glan Clwyd - which turned into a quick
but painful affair. My head didn't pop open and it seems that the
surgeons have all done a fantastic job. My hair is also growing back
quite rapidly (fortunately more or less the same colour too - always a
bonus!) - but anything covering the scar area really irritates me at the
moment, so I'm having to clip my weird 'half hair' back out of the way.

Anyway, after the stitches (ouch, painful - meany nurse) were removed
and I had met with one of the surgeons it was time for surprise
number one! Apparently some big-wig from NHS Wales had popped
in to watch my surgery (blinking heck, the theatre must have been
rather crowded) and is now interested in my case and I was asked if I
minded him coming along to my activation. Of course, I'm all for
sharing the good work of the NHS, so agreed.

A bit funny that even when I am not at work I'm still doing my bit for
the 'patient experience'.

Next it was time for surprise number two - my audiologist wanted to
test the implant, which I wasn't expecting to happen so soon.

Anyway, she rigged my up to the machine and attached the magnet to
my head (weird, but not in a bad way - it gave me the giggles), next she
asked me to say if I heard or felt anything (us deafies feel sound when
it can't be heard).

Differently Human

As there are 22 implant channels each was switched on in turn - and I HEARD a beep/ring sound for every single one!!!!

OK it sounded like an out-of-tune Recorder recital, as played by a five year old - but at least I heard it. It was absolutely bonkers hearing sound inside my head, instead of having the sound blasted at my defunct ear drums. It was a kind of emotional experience.

To top the visit off I was given a H U G E case (to keep, ha ha) full of the implant bits, bobs and gadgets - I love a 'pack' so I'm just steadying myself before I properly unpack it. The funniest thing is that the case looks like a giant iPod! I'm really hoping that I can have some 'show and tell' sessions so that I can show off the goods.

The big 'switch on' will take place on the 30th of December, so yet another countdown now begins.

Number of sleeps since implantation: 9

Today's thoughts: Tiger Mom

We have found out today that my little cub (well 15 year old son) has broken his hand - my goodness, the tiger mom in me would do anything to protect my own children - fortunately little cub (Dear Son) is not in any pain and is positively delirious with happiness that his school year has ended sooner than expected!!

On a lighter note Hubby and I spent the afternoon going through my new toy box - the novelty of sticking the magnet to my head is endlessly amusing - going to try household implements next :)

There is so much to learn; no doubt I'll bore you all with it all in the days to come (when we have worked it out, that is!)

Number of sleeps since implantation: 10

Today's thoughts: Some loveliness to restore Yin and Yang

I have been incredibly spoiled today. My lovely friend took me to John Lewis' to look at all things sparkly (plus to eat cake, drink coffee and indulge in lunch).

More flowers have arrived, my front room (by 'eck - that makes me sound 'reet northern) is now looking to a fantastic flower emporium.

Today's cochlear implant fact!

I can no longer use, or even remotely go near - a Van de Graaf generator (oh the excitement of 3rd Year Physics - making your hair stand on end) - if I did it would do utterly bizarre things to my implant.

Another thing - I now have to carry my cochlear implant ID card at all times - to warn others/security systems/ magnetic fields that I am a cyborg.

"Everything has its wonders, even darkness and silence, and I learn whatever state I am in, therein to be content."

~ Hellen Keller

Differently Human

Number of sleeps since implantation: 11

Today's thoughts: An onion as well as a cyborg

I have an aching skull today. Everyday seems to reveal another layer of ache - perhaps it's the healing working from inside out.

I'm also a bit of a clumsy so-and-so, as I banged my head getting into my car. Fortunately it about 2 inches away from where the implant is - even so it was a bit of a wake-up call about being careful.

Anyway, time for today's cochlear implant fact!

An implant uses binary language (0 and 1) which is then processed by the circuitry inside the implant, which now lives in my skull. This binary language is then converted into signals, which my brain then (well hopefully) makes sense of and learns to interpret as sound.

It's amazing to think that the device which is now melding its way into my humanness has more power than a lot of desktop PCs.

Must dash, visitors have arrived - I hope the weekend is a good one for you :)

Ladies and Gentlemen of the class of '97

Wear sunscreen. If I could offer you only one tip for the future, sunscreen would be it. The long term benefits of sunscreen have been proved by scientists, whereas the rest of my advice has no basis or reliable then my own meandering experience. I will dispense this advice....now.

Enjoy the power and beauty of your youth. Oh, never mind, you won't understand the power and beauty of your youth until they've faded, but trust me in 20 years, you'll look back at photos of yourself and recall in a way you can't grasp now how much possibility lay before you and how fabulous you really looked. You are not as fat as you imagine.

Don't worry about the future, or worry, but know that worrying is as effective as trying to solve an algebra equation by chewing bubblegum.

The real troubles in your life are apt to be things that never crossed your worried mind: the kind that blindsides you at 4pm on some idle Tuesday.

Do one thing every day that scares you.

Sing.

Don't be reckless with other people's hearts; don't put up with people who are reckless with yours.

Floss.

Don't waste your time on jealousy. Sometimes you're ahead, sometimes you're behind. The race is long, and in the end, it's only with yourself.

Remember compliments you receive; forget the insults. (if you succeed in doing this, tell me how).

Keep your old love letters; throw away your old bank statements.

Stretch.

Don't feel guilty if you don't know what you want to do with your life. The most interesting people I know didn't know at 22 what they wanted to do with their lives; some of the most interesting 40 year olds I know still don't.

Get plenty of Calcium. Be kind to your knees - you'll miss them when they're gone.

Maybe you'll marry, maybe you won't. Maybe you'll have children, maybe you won't. Maybe you'll divorce at 40; maybe you'll dance the funky chicken on your 75th wedding anniversary.

Whatever you do, don't congratulate yourself too much or berate yourself, either. Your choices are half chance, so are everybody else's.

Enjoy your body: use it every way you can. Don't be afraid of it or what other people think of it; it's the greatest instrument you'll ever own.

Dance...even if you have nowhere to do it but in your own living room.

Read the directions (even if you don't follow them).

Do not read beauty magazines; they will only make you feel ugly.

Get to know your parents; you never know when they'll be gone for good.

Be nice to your siblings: they're your best link to your past and the people most likely to stick with you in the future.

Understand that friends come and go, but what a precious few should hold on. Work hard to bridge the gaps and geography and lifestyle, because the older you get, the more you need the people you knew when you were young.

Live in New York City once, but leave before it makes you hard.

Live in Northern California once, but leave before it makes you soft.

Travel.

Accept certain inalienable truths: prices will rise, politicians will philander, you too will get old; and when you do, you'll fantasize that when you were young, prices were reasonable, politicians were noble, and children respected their elders.

Respect your elders.

Don't expect anyone else to support you. Maybe you have a trust fund, maybe you'll have a wealthy spouse, but you never know when either one might run out.

Don't mess too much with your hair or by the time you are 40, it will look 85.

Be careful whose advice you buy, but be patient with those who supply it. Advice is a form of nostalgia; dispensing it is a way of wishing the past from the disposal - wiping it off, painting over the ugly parts, and recycling it for more than it's worth.

But trust me, I'm the sunscreen.

~Mary Schmich /Baz Luhrman

Number of sleeps since implantation: 12

Today's thoughts: Odd shape under my skin

The swelling is reducing around the operation site now and I can clearly feel the shape of the implant under my furry head - it is pretty weird. It feels a bit squishy - like the soft part of a baby's head.

It feels weird that this new shape is becoming a part of me... a bit freaky if I think about it too much.

Today's cochlear implant fact!

Insufficient research has been carried out on the effects of Bungee Jumping in implantees - the best they can suggest is that the external components are removed if you want to risk it...don't think I'll be adding to that particular research data base.

Number of sleeps until activation of implant: 10

Today's thoughts: London Calling (very quietly)

Yesterday we ventured to London, as it was our 9 year old Goddaughter's and BIL's Christmas present. As we're big fans of the big city (being rural mice) we decided to give GD and BIL an 'experience' for Christmas. It was also going to be an experience for me too - going to a big, noisy city with just one sort-of functioning ear (or hearing device).

It was a total joy to see London through GD's eyes - which was made even more memorable thanks to the snow in London. Despite the cold we all had a brill time, managing to squeeze in Trafalgar Square, Whitehall, Houses of Parliament, South Bank, Covent Garden, Leicester Square, China Town, Piccadilly Circus and Hyde Park Winter Wonderland into a day! Virgin Trains decided to *give* us a tour of the Midlands on the way home, so our journey ended up taking 4 hours - we eventually got home at 3am...

So London in mono - my first impressions were that it was extremely quiet... Then I realised it was me NOT London. I did feel slightly worried when walking around that I was going to get my head bashed - the implant seems to be very close to the surface of my skin and I have weird visions of it popping out... eeewwww.

Today I have started my countdown to implant activation (aka - learning to be deaf in a different way).

I have read many stories about activation day and it seems that to start with I will hear a cross between Donald Duck, Daleks and Miss. Othmar (from the Peanuts cartoon). My brain will have to start habituating the sound to sound like what I think things sound like... it's so complicated

London calling, yes, I was there, too   An' you know what they said? Well, some of it was true!   London calling at the top of the dial   And

after all this, won't you give me a smile?   London Calling   I never felt
so much alive, alive, alive...

~ The Clash

Number of sleeps until activation of implant: 9

Today's thoughts: Too many to narrow it down

A big day for me, re-visiting my workplace, have I changed?

Has it changed? Not really but yes (which probably makes no sense
whatsoever...)

I must admit my stomach really churned on the short drive to my
workplace. Thankfully, my wonderfully thoughtful friend met me at the
door and walked me through the building to our office (I'd possibly
have been standing there now if she hadn't).

The first thing I noticed was how quiet it was, not that it was actually
quiet, but hearing through one ear made everywhere seem ultra silent -
even though I could see people chattering away around me. My team
were as kind as ever - we seem to share the same ironic sense of
humour which helps (and yes we can try attaching paperclips to my
head!!!)

After an hour I really felt tired, I hadn't really accounted for the fact
that hearing outside my house is doubly tiring when in mono -
something I will have be mindful of - one step at a time, as I was
reminded today!

This afternoon Hubby and I visited Bridgemere Garden World on our mission to visit all of the garden centres in our locality. It was really quiet (yes, quiet *quiet*) so we enjoyed a mooch, plus fortifying slice of carrot cake.

Today's cochlear implant fact!

An implant has 22 electrodes which attempt to generate sound. These 22 electrodes work in combination to create the tone, pitch etc. The human ear has approximately 3,500 inner ear hair cells, which work together to create sound.

I think this fact brings home the reality comparison of what an implant may achieve compared to 'normal' hearing.

However, I am very grateful to have this opportunity to try.

Number of sleeps until activation of implant: 8

Today's thoughts: Ouch, tired - need some light at the end of my tunnel

Hmmm... another visit to work and another realisation of just how demanding sound and concentrating is. It makes everything seem a little insurmountable at times. I am so fortunate that people DO seem to be interested and I'm sure that I will get a lot of support on my return - the hardest part for me will be actually letting people help.

At work we shared lunch as a team, although I put my 'being positive' face on, I did feel rather lost. Thankfully the tomato incident did cheer me up no end!!!

My scar is really uncomfortable today too (maybe that's what making me a grouch). I have put the steroid tape on to try and speed up the healing, but it hasn't had any effect this time. Also Hubby has informed me that there appears to me some white cotton sticking out of the scar... maybe it's from the underneath stitches.

Number of sleeps until activation of implant: 7

Today's thoughts: The sound of silence

I think I might have mentioned that I am currently reading a book called 'Rebuilt' by Michael Chorost. It follows the author's story of being implanted (in America about 10 or so years ago).

How I wish I had come across this book before - all the time when I really, genuinely did think I was losing my mind, I was actually going through a fairly normal transition. Pretty much every word written rings true for me. Here is a short paragraph about the period before the author's implantation:

> **But most of all I have become an emotional creature I can't recognise. I'm sobbing in my car, sobbing in locked bathrooms, sobbing on my couch at home. To be sure, anyone would grieve for lost ears and fear an uncertain future, but these feeling are like a jagged slash torn in the beige fabric of my life.**

I certainly recognise myself there; I expect those who know me would too.

The flip side of this, for me personally, is trying to come to terms with what I am now - gosh I sound so bloody self indulgent - but trust me on this one - it is a real challenge.

I am definitely going to put together information for the hospital (Glan Clwyd) for adults undergoing the cochlear implantation process, particularly for young (!) adults who have become deafened. Hopefully my psychology studies will help. I desperately want something positive from my experiences to be helpful to others in the future.

On a lighter note - as it is the eve, of Christmas Eve (as my Dear Daughter would say!!) the shopping marathon is now complete - if I haven't bought it, I certainly won't be buying it tomorrow :)

I'm still waiting for my Hubby's presents to be delivered from Amazon (they should have arrived on the 8th of December - it appears that Royal Mail sent the parcel to Scotland and it's been stuck in the snow ever since) - so I am going to have to be creative if they don't arrive tomorrow.

And another thing - I managed to pull out the white piece of cotton from my scar! It was an inch long, eeewwww - totally freaky :)

Number of sleeps until activation of implant: 6

Today's thoughts: Silent Night

Just a word of thanks to those who have/are following my cochlear implant journey - my stats tell me readers from the UK, USA, Croatia, Malaysia and Singapore have joined the ride.

Thinking of Christmas, the best 'gift' we can hope to give to others and receive from others is that of understanding.

Sometimes it's so complicated to make sense of our own lives, never mind others - but trying to understand and walk alongside someone is the best gift of all - it doesn't cost us a penny either.

I hope this Christmas brings you many smiles.

Number of sleeps until activation of implant: 5

Today's thoughts: When I'm in the crowd.

I hope this day is bringing you good cheer.

It's been a slightly different day in the Leigh Household, due to changes in our family set-up, plus Dear Daughter announced her engagement!

Apart from the obligatory burnt digit, we have had a relaxing day - I have purposefully decided to keep our family gatherings small this year, so I can at least feel involved in things - my BIGGEST bug bear as a deafy is social gatherings, as I feel 'outside the bubble' - watching stuff happening, I wonder if that will change when the implant is switched on.

When I'm in the crowd, I can't remember my name and my only link is pots of Wall's ice cream when I'm in the crowd - I don't see anything

~ The Jam

Number of sleeps until activation of implant: 4

Today's thoughts: Out with the old...

Another round of family gatherings to contend with/enjoy today.

For some reason, my Mother decided to 'share' her new violin concert DVD with us. At the best of times it would sound bad - but with one hearing aid and background chatter to me it sounded like rush hour traffic (or at least what I think rush hour traffic sounds like!).

We then popped to visit various in-laws and more noise confusion reigned, in the end it seemed easier to sit there with an enigmatic smile on my face.

Just returned home to make curry out of the beef leftovers - nothing at all to do with having a cochlear implant - but at least you know how I have spent my Boxing Day :)

Number of sleeps until activation of implant: 3

Today's thoughts: Parallel worlds

The bizarre joys of being a deaf person were brought home to me this afternoon in quite unique circumstances!

After Hubby and I took Dear Daughter and her Fiancé home to Sale, we decided to take the scenic route (the M6 was going at a snail's pace) - and stopped off at a Garden Centre (obviously still on our quest to visit Cheshire's finest!!)

As with all our visits to garden centres our first stop was the coffee shop. We placed out order and then began chatting about a TV programme I had watched earlier about Indian Railways (yes I know, strange) - I'm definitely going to save up to visit as soon as funds allow.

Anyway the drinks arrived and we carried on our conversation.

Hubby: So what do you like about *muffled*

Me: Sorry, say that again, what do I like about what??

Hubby: *finger spells the muffled word*

Me: In here? Well I like the tasty food and the interesting gift shop on the way out!

Hubby: Ehhh? No, INDIA - what do you like about INDIA?

Cue lots of spluttering and laughing! I thought Hubby had said, 'what do you like about in here' - meaning the garden centre :)

So in my alternative reality the conversation went, so Emma, what do you like India?

"Because of its tasty food and the interesting gift shop on the way out!"

Ha ha, it is still making me laugh now :)

For the record, I like INDIA for the culture, amazing scenery etc! (However, I'm sure the food is also good and there are plenty of interesting gift shops!!!)

Number of sleeps until activation of implant: 2

Today's thoughts: It's all a bit of a jumble really

Woke up feeling dizzy again today AND another two white stitches have appeared, one which has fallen out (makes me wonder if I am coming apart at the seams on the inside - ahhh, the irony).

Feeling a little anxious about the 'switch on' - as I have spent the last three weeks becoming acclimatised to being a person with one functioning ear (well hearing aid in my case).

I have tried on the head gear... errr.. processor again, and this time I didn't like it so much. I suppose I had better LEARN to like it as its going to be my new constant companion.

Perhaps I should give it a name to make it seem some personable?? Maybe Ludwig after Beethoven!

> A cyborg is seen as a person who is "differently human" by becoming, to some degree, directly dependent on technology/software for life-enhancing or life-preserving functions, i.e. - a cochlear implantee.

Number of sleeps until activation of implant: 1

Today's thoughts: What if I don't like it???

Taken down the Christmas decorations today, as it seemed right that as I had put them up just before the operation, they needed to come down before switch on - the new beginning...

I have been faffing around with the processor today, trying to 'pair' it up with the remote assistant, so that they talk to each other (useful for when I want to alter the volume, change the programmes, switch it on and off etc).

It was pretty complicated, I think I'll be walking around with the instruction book for a while, working out what the different coloured flashes mean.

From tomorrow onwards, these will be my constant companions, wherever I go, Ludwig (yep, I've settled on Ludwig for my processors name) will accompany me.

Part of me still thinks, what did I do to end up here, in this situation, kinda thing... karma works in funny ways I guess.

My brother has also kindly brought me a talking book (CD and verbatim book) to assist with my initial word recognition.

My audiologist recommends that I start of children's books as they have simpler sentences and language. So my first book is officially.... Finding Nemo!!

Number of sleeps until activation of implant: still 1

Feeling really anxious and can't settle................................ :(

Number of sleeps until activation of implant: 0 - Today's the day

Not sure that I can even begin describing today, it has been the strangest day ever...

Here is a summary.

Arrived at hospital and introduced to Chief Exec chap.

Rigged up to the computer by Dr. Marie - hearing aid removed.

Another test of the electrodes to check that they are still firing - they were.

The moment of truth, the big switch on by Dr. Marie..... a slight pause... cue lots of strange bleeps and whirrs (imagine the sound of being 'beamed' somewhere in Star Trek/Wars) another pause, then a strange tinny voice saying, 'can you hear me? Tell me if you hear anything?'

I then burst into laughter as it sounded like I was being addressed by a mixture of Mickey Mouse, R2D2 and C-P30 - the 'big moment' and all I could do was giggle :D

We all then sat around marvelling at how wonderful the human brain is, while I continued to giggle...

A short break for a brew, then I met the hearing therapist, who put me through my paces to determine where the rehab needs to start.

Bizarrely I ACED all the tests; I have never concentrated so hard in my life! She and Hubby were really amazed (me too - I was being very serious at this point) - I must point out that my responses are the exception to the rule; people don't normally recite sentences after just an hour of wearing an implant.

Elaine the hearing therapist then took me on an 'environmental tour' to listen to doors, air conditioning, toilets flushing(!!!) and such like, weird - I never realised these things makes noises. I'm also going to have to start tip toeing about, I sound like a fairy elephant clomping around.

After lunch we concentrated on setting up my remote assistant, which is now known as Ludwig 2. I now have a variety of programmes to try before my next appointment in 7 days time.

It is fair to say I am absolutely exhausted now; my brain is well and truly frazzled - which is normal.

Think I am going to have to take a fold up bed wherever I go then I can have a nap - goodness only knows how I am going to get on when I go back to work.

Days since activation of implant: 1

New sounds: None yet, as I haven't got Ludwig out of the box...

By the end of the day yesterday my brain stopped recognising sounds and the sound level from the implant dropped significantly (I was warned that this would happen). In typical deafy fashion, I just wanted it to be **LOUDER** and **LOUDER**.

Well, it's the first new day of my 'other' deaf life.

I'm feeling more emotional about the experience today, the excitement of yesterday has given way to feeling a little more anxious today (thank goodness for the miracle of happy pills).

The new sounds that I heard yesterday are so vastly different to what I have heard before, even what I think I can remember hearing before. It is so strange having the sensation of sound **inside** my head instead of it blasting at my ear drums. It's almost as if I can feel the sensation of the electrodes firing off. Another thing I noticed is that there is a very, very slight delay in the sound registering - which I suppose is understandable, given that the processors need to do their work.

Hubby thinks that my new head gear is cool - given that he is quite a fan of the Six Million Dollar Man, he now has his very own Cyborg.

Anyway, I expect I'm going to have to bite the proverbial bullet and get Ludwig out now...

Days since activation of implant: 2

New sounds: The clock 'ticks' in my front room

Firstly - a very happy, healthy, kind, motivating, wish fulfilling New Year to you dear readers - if you have ever wanted to do something new, let this be the year that you do it. Without sounding cheesy, every day really does count (and don't forget to wear some sparkles, your best frocks and to burn your fancy candles).

I DO hope that you can continue on this journey with me - it feels a little scary at the moment, so the more riders in the train, the better.

I was reminded yesterday that no matter what, my 'hearing condition' was for life anyway (believe me - it is one 'present' I'd had gladly given back) - so in essence I have replaced one lifelong condition with something else - the implant - which is still a condition I'll have to work around in some shape or form, plus without the implant I'm now even more profoundly deaf than ever :(

While I might be coming across as a grumpy, ungrateful cow at the moment, I apologise, the whole issue with losing my hearing continues to be an *issue* for me.

Anyway, I'll slap on my positive face - you'll be glad to know that I lasted pretty much all day with the processor on yesterday, it's not uncomfortable to wear and to be honest I can hardly tell I'm wearing it for most of the time. The magnetic coil is actually quite cosy, though the implant site itself is quite swollen still.

It is nice not having a load of plastic squished in my ear too. Incidentally the wonderfully kind people at Glan Clwyd gave me something called a 'drying box' to take the moisture out of both my processor and hearing aid {it's a bit like a tumble dryer for hearing devices!!}. It is a **BRILLIANT** gadget, for the first time ever my poor stinky hearing aid has actually felt clean and fresh, which will hopefully reduce the number of ear infections that I get. It does make me wonder why the English NHS don't provide these - think of all the money they would save on antibiotics.

Anyway, when I'm sitting in the quiet of my front room, I can hear my mantle clock ticking, which Hubby tells me is actually very quiet indeed. When others are talking I can't hear it, but then again, people with good hearing wouldn't necessarily hear it either. Environmental sounds are easier to understand than speech so far, as their tones are usually quite deep and in one pitch.

When I went to bed last night, I had the strangest bout of tinnitus ever; it was like two cats screeching at each other. My poor brain was obviously trying to suck sound from somewhere... perhaps it was missing Ludwig!

Days since activation of implant: 3

New sounds: Hubby playing the guitar badly (while he is upstairs and I am downstairs)

My head is still buzzing from all the new information that Ludwig is providing me, it gets a bit much sometimes and I have to yank the damn thing off (carefully, obviously).

Something that I didn't prepare myself for is the new additions to my daily regime.

In the morning I have to switch everything on, then check the battery (which is a rechargeable) to see if it has enough power for the day (more noise requires more battery power as the processor needs to work harder).

I then have to put my other battery to charge on its recharging dock.

Following this I then switch my remote control (Ludwig 2) on, to alter the hearing environment, if required, and to do the 'is everything working OK' check.

At night the whole process is reversed, but Ludwig has to be placed in the drying out box. I have four different chargers and plugs for all these gadgets...

I came across an Australian blog yesterday of a woman called Katie who has done a blog about the process of receiving a cochlear implant. Weirdly we have both written about almost identical things - which makes who feel a little more normal thankfully.

Katie had also written in depth about the isolation of deafness, personally I don't think those feelings will ever truly go away - at least with the implant it shows that we are willing to try pretty much anything (after all, given the choice would you willingly choose to walk around with a magnet and wires sticking to your head for the rest of your life??) to be accepted and included in the hearing world.

There's now only one day until I am due back at work, which I am dreading. The last four weeks seem to have sapped what confidence I had. While the work won't really have changed too much, I have.

Days since activation of implant: 4

New sounds: Dear Son chattering on his mobile phone in the kitchen, where he thinks I can't hear him (no more hiding from Mummy, ha ha!!)

I'm going to apologise before I continue, as this one is going to get pretty graphic. In fairness to the cochlear implant journey I am going to have to detail the nocturnal events which are happening.

As mentioned previously, Ludwig my processor gets switched off and put into its drying case for the evening. Last night I fancied a bit of a read, so took a book up to bed with me. After an hour or so I felt tired, so put my book down and turned off the lights (Hubby was dozing away merrily at this point).

Anyway, I switched off the light and got back into bed (this was about midnight), then it started - the white noise.

This noise is a new take on tinnitus (I have suffered from tinnitus for years, but this is really something else). The minute I try to relax and go to sleep the noise begins. Last night it sounded like the warbled sounds of a guitar playing (was it my brain trying to keep a grasp of what it had heard in the day??). It then turned to screeches and the hiss of white noise. Believe me, it sounds so loud to me I want to YELL loudly for it to SHUT UP. Part of me wanted to smash my head against the wall to make the sounds stop, it was pure torture.

For the next FOUR hours, I tossed, turned, sat up, lay back down, put my head under the pillow, propped my head up with more pillows to try and make it go away. In seriousness I considered getting up and swigging a bottle of Night Nurse or something to knock myself out. The last time I looked at my clock it was 4.31am...

I eventually woke up at just before 10am, which doesn't bode well for getting up for work tomorrow. I currently feel like crap. I'm really hoping that at my mapping appointment on Thursday I can be given some useful strategies to manage it :(

Days since activation of implant: 5

New sounds: Arghhhh... keyboards

It's pretty difficult knowing what to say today...

Anyway, it's my first day (or to be accurate, part day) back at work - I feel like my head has been replaced by a cabbage.

It was so easy to slip back into the routine of being 'positive me' - even when I am feeling pretty void inside.

Weirdly, I have got used to wearing Ludwig the processor and have accepted the benefits of the implant (heck, I'm even happy that I have had the operation done), but when I go back into a regular domain, like my workplace I feel a bit like a freak (hmmm... seems like I still have some work to do).

Thankfully my return to work is a phased one - which I need more than I thought I did - 5 hours today felt like a marathon (or maybe it was the never ending stream of emails to go through). Hopefully it will get easier.

Even though it was a quiet day at the office today, there were lots of new sounds for me... I never realised typing on keyboards was so loud - I always thought they were silent :) The sandwich vans, which visit our workplace, also have loud horns/tunes when they arrive - I have wondered in the past why people all seemed to get up together and disappear!

Later…

I think I'm losing my mind....

I decided to take Ludwig off a little earlier today as it has been a big day and I've had lots of new sounds to deal with (I also ended up having to charge everything up this afternoon too - flashing lights and bleeps a plenty telling me to take action).

I also had an ulterior motive that by taking the processor off earlier, then the white noise might stop earlier too.

IT'S NOT BLINKING WELL WORKED :(

The more I try to ignore it, the louder it gets, hiss hiss hiss, twang twang twang, then a power drill kind of noise....

My choices:

Scream and try and drown out the noise

Rant - but no one's home only me (well I could rant here...)

Put the bloody processor back on again... nooooo...

Rummage in cupboards to see if we have any Kalms, Nytol and take the blinking lot...

It's going to be a long night....

Days since activation of implant: 6

New sounds: Fire alarm at work

Today has not been a great success - reminders of why I don't belong. I'm a freak and a fool to think I did. The cochlear implant has succeeded in changing me, but not changing a thing.

Quote from Helen Keller ~

The problems of deafness are deeper and more complex, if not more important than those of blindness. Deafness is a much worse misfortune. For it means the loss of the most vital stimulus-- the sound of the voice that brings language, sets thoughts astir, and keeps us in the intellectual company of man. Blindness separates us from things but deafness separates us from people.

I hope dear readers that you have had a better day.

Tesco throws me a few crumbs of comfort

You know what it's like; you are having a lousy day - wondering why you bothered getting out of bed...

It seems that Tesco is now my number one provider of entertainment :) Yes, that's a smile - first one today.

I popped in to buy a few bits and bobs and made my way to the self-service till to pay (easier than having to deal with checkout staff....)

Anyway, I put my goods through, bleep bleep bleep, then pressed 'finish and pay'.

Then instead of the usual deep and sultry tones of, 'please swipe your clubcard,' it was a squeaky high-pitched Minnie Mouse version, 'please swipe your clubcard'!!!

Cue Emma looking around to see if anyone else was finding the voice as funny as me!!!

The cochlear implant changes the voice of **ANYTHING** which has a voice!!

I can see that Ludwig and the self-service checkout are going to become firm friends :)

Days since activation of implant: 7

New sounds: Perfume squirting, prfft

Good job I had requested annual leave for this morning (before my 2nd mapping appointment) as I woke up to see Dear Son off to school then promptly fell asleep for another two hours - all the extra brain activity is wearing me out. Still feeling rather 'winded' after yesterday, even Hubby noticed that I seem to have gone backwards...

Anyway, it was quite a relief to go back to Glan Clwyd as it feels kinda safe there; with people who make me feel normal and accepted.

My first appointment was with Elaine the hearing therapist who did some tests on my consonant recognition. Consonant recognition is more difficult than vowel recognition as they often don't have a 'sound' associated with them (practice saying 'a' - ahhh, then saying 'p' - puh).

I pleased to say I did well. Elaine said that I am continuing to make her job easier as I don't really need any rehab from her, just to go about my normal day to day stuff and let the sounds sink in.

After a short break (yes, the sessions include breaks as they are pretty exhausting), I met with Dr. Marie who did some speech recognition tests, to check my progress at week one. The speech tests involve listening to a round of 25 sentences, first with just the implant, then both hearing aid and implant together. This is then followed by individual word discrimination. The sentences are really random, so you can't guess as them, things like: the girl argues with her sister and the strawberry jam is very sweet.

> **My scores:**
>
> **Pre-implant, left ear (which is now implanted ear) ➜ 49% on sentence recognition**
>
> **Post-implant, left side ➜ 77% on sentence recognition**
>
> **Post implant, using both implant and hearing aid ➜ 85% on sentence recognition**
>
> **Pre-implant, left ear ➜ 0% on individual word recognition**
>
> **Post-implant, left side ➜ 27% on individual word recognition**

All in all this is really outstanding after just a week!

I was so pleased so get such good results as it feels like I'm giving something back to those who have invested their time and energy in me. Dr. Marie was also kind enough to say how everyone has enjoyed working with me as I try so hard and am good at following the rather extensive instructions!

Dr. Marie also did another sound map with me, checking my thresholds and the like - so in effect it's like my brain has been given a new road map to follow, just when it was beginning to find its way with the old one (well it should make for an interesting bout of tinnitus later).

Days since activation of implant: 8

New sounds: The telephone ringing in my hall

Well somehow I survived the week - discovered some new stuff, been reminded of the old stuff. It's been a week of odd reactions to say the least...

I can certainly tell a difference between the sound maps, and it does feels I have maybe taken a step backwards in the learning process today.

I DO think that I and everyone around me need to remember that having the cochlear implant is NOT a cure for deafness, it's just like having a hearing aid embedded in your head (Carla my implantee buddy's words - not mine, she has got her head around things much better than me).

Obviously the long-term hope is that things like lip reading will become easier and less tiring. As Elaine the hearing therapist said yesterday, "it's only been 7 days out of a life time; give yourself a break."

Well I'm having a break at the moment as Hubby and Dear Son are having a jamming session. Since I had a horrendous bout of tinnitus which sounded like garbled guitars I am sitting here minus my hearing devices - which feels like I have switched my brain off too!

Days since activation of implant: 9

New sounds: My daughter's voice (we've not seen each other since Christmas, so it was the first time I had heard her voice using the implant)

Today was a lesson that I need to be more prepared.

I met up with my Dear Daughter to go shopping for a new guinea pig today (for her not me - I don't have space for another cage!!) and we had a lovely afternoon mooching around the shops and eventually choosing a new piggy.

We then collected Hubby and returned to Sale to drop off Dear Daughter and piggy (plus various piggy goodies).

After 10 minutes or so of chatting, I got the series of dreaded bleeps telling me that my battery was about to go flat. Unfortunately I didn't have a spare with me, so had to switch off - well actually I got a series of very indignant bleeps and the processor switched itself off!

Immediately I was shunted straight back outside the bubble - although DD and Hubby didn't exclude me, I could no longer keep up with the conversation (which goes to show how quickly I am becoming reliant on Ludwig).

We returned home and I have put everything to charge once again. I'm definitely going to have to be better prepared and carry around a charged up spare, or the kit which allows me to use some disposables (sounds like I am going to need a bigger bag...).

Days since activation of implant: 10

New sounds: Metallica at Milton Keynes Bowl, circa 1993, courtesy of YouTube

Me and Hubby have been having a blast from the past today and have been busy searching out concert footage, from when we were kids - well kids with kids!

Bizarrely my implant picks up quite well from my PC speakers, so we have been reliving the greats of Metallica, Megadeath, The Almighty, Diamond Head, Guns and Roses and The Cult.

In case anyone is wondering, no my hearing loss wasn't caused by listening to loud music at concerts...

It has been good to have some access to sounds from my past, it's things like that which help to reinforce my identity - who I was then, who I am now etc.

Days since activation of implant: 11

New sounds: Trying to keep up with multiple voices

A real back to reality day today, with three work meetings, one after the other.

It is the first time I have been involved with a large meeting since I returned last week, so keeping up with the Dalek voices was a little unusual to say the least! Weirdly my brain keep fluctuating between implant and hearing aid - it couldn't seem to make its mind up which was it was going to concentrate on. Anyway, it was good to feel involved and it was nice to be welcomed back - crikey, have I actually been missed??!!

Days since activation of implant: 12

New sounds: Announcements on the train

Today feels like it has been a t least three weeks long.

I went to bed early last night as I knew I would have a busy day today working in Manchester.

In order to distract myself from the horrid white noise I read for a while, well until I was doing the thing when your book keeps falling out of your hands but you carry on reading regardless.

Things were looking good - I had a quick chat to Hubby (no implant and no hearing aids either, I'm pretty good at lip reading him!) and turned the light off quickly - it was 10.30pm.

Then the noise started, the second my brain stopped concentrating on anything. For half an hour I lay in bed, trying just about every relaxation exercise I know - but it didn't work, so I got up and made hot chocolate and had an extra happy pill for relaxation purposes (I'm desperate OK).

After watching a bit of TV I felt a bit drowsy so I went back to bed quickly - only to find the minute I lay down the noise re-started. (Midnightish by now). In total exasperation I got up and put my implant back on - but the noise continued and merrily amplified the ticking of my clock, so Ludwig was sent to solitary confinement in the drying box.

I then watched Shameless (fab) and Homes Under the Hammer (!!!!) before eventually nodding off at 3am.

I was up again at 6am, desperate not to miss my train into Manchester.

This whole tinnitus business is a real massive downside to the implant, which I'm becoming increasing fond of.

Days since activation of implant: 13

New sounds: The door into my workplace really creaks - how can I have possibly have missed that?

A slightly better night's sleep last night, I did manage to SLEEP until 3am, and then woke up - so a bit of a back to front night.

Carla my implantee buddy experienced the same after her implant, so hopefully I will grow out of it too - it seems my head has turned into a new born baby!

So sideways glances - I happened to notice some sideways glances from people today, obviously trying to work out what it is I have stuck to my head. It seems that people are splitting into two groups - those who seem really interested about the implant, wanting to know how it works etc; and those who freak out at the sight of the implant (my TWIN brother was one of those, when he first looked at the implant he grimaced, like he was looking at a rancid, gaping wound).

Days since activation of implant: 14

New sounds: Too much new noise

It's been a day of the doldrums today; I think it must be contagious as we all seem to have it at work.

The day started off with a few pointed questions from a fairly 'distant' colleague, who then informed me my voice is changing - though another Dear Colleague in the background was shaking her head!!!!

Perhaps I was using my posh voice :)

I was also asked if the magnet was a permanent fixture, or was it detachable, which is kinda funny I suppose. Well actually they do make bone anchored implants, where they make a sort of permanent plug in your head that you then attach a small box too - eeewwww imagine having a 'port' on your head - that is really a step too weird even for me.

I am now well accustomed to actually wearing Ludwig the processor, it is much more comfortable than a hearing aid - the massive plus side is not having my ear bunged up with plastic all the time.

As the doldrums day continued all the new noise started to get a bit too much, my brain is still at the stage where it is trying to take on board everything it hears, its 'not relevant filter' hasn't kicked in yet.

My Dear Colleague sitting next to me even informed me that I was being too loud, bashing away at my keyboard (I am now aware that I type rather LOUDLY... - whoops, sorry Dear Colleagues)

Days since activation of implant: 15

Hello Dear Readers.

Today is going to be my last entry in my implantation diary.

As far as my cochlear implant journey goes, there isn't really much new to report each day - me telling you about sounds you are familiar with is NOT such exciting reading!

I thought I'd sum up the whole experience (to date) so that if any of you are thinking about an implant for yourself or a member of your family you have my opinion - like it or not :)

So here goes!

Before

Make sure that your audiologist gives you the choice of where you will be treated, and check out your options. I am really pleased I chose

Glan Clwyd - they have been marvellous, treating me like a human being with thoughts, ideas and feelings at all times.

Try and find a buddy (if you are lucky like me your hospital will help). Getting to know Carla was really important to me (when if I did come across as having a hair fixation). No one really understands like someone who has also walked down the same path, wearing the same shoes. I'm lucky now in that I have a friend for life in Carla.

Talk. What I mean is, don't bottle things up. Even if you just manage to tell people that you feel scared, say it.

Make sure that you fully research different implant manufacturers (not all implants are the same). Try and find one that will work for YOU in YOUR life.

Lean on your friends and family. In my case my wider family just weren't there. My friends have been invaluable - they have shown me such kindness and understanding, even when I was at my most manic.

My own immediate family - Hubby, Dear Son and Dear Daughter have been, and continue to be amazing.

During (surgery)

Rest - it's pretty major having your head unzipped.

Sleep as much as you can.

Don't be embarrassed about your bald head - show it off with pride - it's one of the few times you can get away with a really wacky hairdo :)

After (switch on)

Expect the unexpected - everybody's experiences are different. Mine was amusing, some people's emotional.

Be realistic - it DOES sound very different from anything you have ever heard before.

Give yourself a break, if you have had years of deafness it WILL take time to get used to using your brain in a different way.

Don't be embarrassed about wearing your implant - it is cool head gear for special people! AND don't let other people make you feel embarrassed either - they are the ones with the issue.

Learn relaxation techniques, on the off chance you develop tinnitus - every little helps.

So that's it. It has been a really useful experience for me to write each day - I can look back on the last two months and feel proud of myself for taking such a big step.

You never know - we might find ourselves back here in the future with Emma's Cochlear Implant Journey - Part Two (but I guess that's another story!!)

That's all from me Dear Readers,

Emma xxxx

Now Ludwig and I are One

Whooo - hello - time flies and all that.

Somehow it seemed appropriate to put fingers to keyboard to make reference to the fact that Ludwig is due to celebrate its first birthday.... I'm one year on from implantation.

So..... what is the biggest 'hearing' difference in a year living with my implant? Environmental sounds - I had forgotten that they existed... the sound of pegs as they clip onto the washing line, taps running (though I still don't react to the sound and leave the sink to overflow...), background chatter (though I still can't make out all of what is being said, I get the semblance of words spoken). Yes lip-reading is easier and I don't always have to follow people's faces (at least people who I know well) so much - but the bottom line is I am still a deaf person, albeit in a different way.

I remember that I received an award just before the operation last year - well I have gone on to be awarded this year's version of that same award - so my brain must be functioning OK! I've also gone on to do a slightly different job - so having the implant has not been a hindrance or a barrier in a work sense. The only issue I could say about the workplace is that people seem to think a cochlear implant is a miracle cure - NOPE - I'm still deaf and I still fall asleep during meetings.

Casting my mind back, the biggest concern I had (apart from having my hair shaved off - ironic in that I DO have short hair now by choice) - was that would I ever be ME again? Hmmmm.... to tell the truth I don't think I can answer that one honestly - I still have ongoing identity issues that plague me... I still don't associate myself with the photos taken of me before the operation, it does seem that person has gone - I feel more brittle now (which certainly doesn't make any sense). I think that possibly I am acting out the person who I think I am. Well it took time for me to accept my deafness in the first place, so I suppose it will take time to accept the new version of me now.

So would I go back and NOT have the implant?

Absolutely NOT - it was the totally right thing for me to do at that time. If I was to be offered an implant for my other ear (which incidentally is practically useless, even with a hearing aid) - I would jump at the chance. Weird pluses include the comfort of wearing the implant compared to a hearing aid - it may look rather freaky but it vastly reduces the number of ear infections.

Of course, there have been challenging times on many occasions this year. The numerous scalp and implant site infections (plus turbo antibiotics, creams and being banned from wearing my implant for a week - the equivalent of being put into solitary confinement); the mapping sessions and getting my brain acclimatised to new hearing road maps; the day-to-day practicalities of being charged up, having spare batteries available, asking people to 'hold that thought' whilst you fumble around trying to rig yourself up again. The tinnitus remains horrendous...

So, that's a whistle stop tour of where 365 days takes you with a cochlear implant - Happy Birthday Ludwig.

Cochlear Implants – some stuff you might want to know

Here is a collection of information about the cochlear implant process. Whilst I can't take any credit for any of this information, it is what I managed to collect after souring the internet.

It is not intended to replace any medical advice whatsoever, plus things seem to change within the world of cochlear implantation, so your implant team will be the best people to explain what happens at their centre.

General information

A cochlear implant is an electronic device which may be suitable for children and adults who receive no useful benefit from conventional hearing aids. Conventional hearing aids work by making sounds louder. A cochlear implant is different because sounds are turned into tiny electrical pulses, which are sent directly to the nerve of hearing. The implant can therefore bypass some of the inner ear structures which are not working. Naturally it is important to remember that no electronic device can be expected to restore function to the levels experienced by a normally hearing ear.

A cochlear implant has several different parts, some of which are internal (cannot be seen) and some of which are external (worn outside the body).

The external components - (worn outside the body)

These look very similar to a body-worn hearing aid, but actually work quite differently. They consist of a microphone, a sound processor and an external transmitter coil, with cables to connect them.

With a cochlear implant, the microphone is placed either behind the ear, like a hearing aid. Cables connect the microphone to the speech processor.

The microphone picks up incoming sounds and changes them into electrical signals, which are then taken down via the long cable to the processor (which is worn behind the ear). The processor contains the batteries which power the entire cochlear implant, and these must be recharged daily. During programming sessions, the processor will have been carefully set to make the signal just right. The signal is then sent back up the long lead, and then to the external transmitter coil and magnet. This looks like a light-weight plastic disc or circle, with the magnet in the middle. The signal passes through the skin using radio waves to meet the internal parts of the implant.

The internal components - (under the skin)

These are the parts of the device implanted by the surgeon during the cochlear implant operation. They include the internal receiver/ stimulator package (with the internal magnet). It lies under the skin behind the ear, and can be felt if touched gently.

The receiver/ stimulator package picks up the radio signal from the outside transmitter coil.

From here, the signal is taken via a thin wire to the cochlea (inner ear). The end of the wire (called the electrode array) is threaded into the cochlea by the surgeon. Because the shape of the cochlea is a spiral (like a tiny snail's shell), inserting the electrode array requires considerable delicacy and skill.

On the electrode array itself, there are several points at which the electrical signals are delivered, these are called the electrodes. The different electrodes each take a part of the signal (depending on whether a particular electrode is tuned for high or low pitches), so that different sounds can stimulate different areas in the cochlea. The signal from the electrodes activates the nerve of hearing, which then takes the message along the usual pathway to the brain. At this stage, the signal may be interpreted by the brain as "a sound".

Experience and practice helps people to begin to tell the difference between some of the sounds the implant is giving them. Obviously this will take a lot of work, and this is where the re/habilitation team will be able to assist and support you,

The Operation
Before the operation, you will be given a general anaesthetic. After which the hair behind the ear is shaved in an area about four inches

from your hairline. The operation takes place in theatre and will take between two and five hours to complete, but normally, in straightforward cases, it will take approximately two hours. You will wake up with a large bandage (like a turban) on your head.

24 - 48 hours later this will be changed for a small dressing. There will be a pack in your ear canal which should be left for a week to protect the wound. A follow up surgery appointment in Outpatients usually takes place about one week after the operation where the ear pack is removed and the scar is checked.

Recovery

Recovery after the operation is variable but most patients feel better very quickly. Most patients do not suffer significant pain after the operation. You are required to check into the ward the day before surgery and you will remain in hospital for one to two nights after the surgery. We recommend that you take two weeks rest at home. Once your hair has grown back and your scar has healed, the only evidence of the operation will be a small bump just behind the ear.

Risks and side effects

A cochlear implant operation carries the same slight risk as other ear surgery. You should, however, be aware of the following possible side effects:-

- The risks associated with having a general anaesthetic

- Temporary dizziness and/or temporary disturbance of balance

- Temporary increase in tinnitus

- Numbness in area of scar

- Change in taste sensation

- A risk of infection

- Facial nerve bruising: This nerve running near the site of surgery is carefully monitored throughout the operation. This ensures that bruising of the facial nerve is highly unlikely.

- The possibility of implant breakdown in the future, in which case a further operation would be necessary to replace it.

- Because the operation is relatively new, the long term effects of electrical stimulation are not known. The amount of electricity involved however, is minimal and during the past fifteen years in which people have received cochlear implants there have been no indications of long term damage.

If you are particularly concerned about any of the above risks you should discuss them with one of the doctors.

Post operation

While you are on the ward one of the nursing staff will show you how to wash your face whilst at the same time protecting the scar area. You are encouraged to wait a minimum of two weeks after surgery before washing your hair. You need to take care to keep the wound dry and be very gentle with that area for the first month. After the first month, treat the wound as normal and if you are a keen swimmer you can restart then. Flying should be avoided for four weeks following surgery.

If required you will be given painkillers on the ward and some to take home.

The surgeon will generally use dissolvable stitches, which do not need to be removed. The area around the scar, including part of your ear, will be numb and sensation will slowly return over a period of six months. However, this may never return fully to normal. You may also have some swelling around your ear, which should settle within the first two to three weeks.

Taking care of yourself
We advise you to avoid all activities that might cause a blow to the head, e.g. rugby, football and boxing as these could potentially cause damage to the implant. Also, we would advise against doing such activities as scuba diving as the pressure changes involved in deep water diving could damage the implant.

The Rehabilitation Process
When a person is beginning to think about cochlear implantation, it is natural to focus on the assessment and surgery phases of the process. However it is important to remember that following these there is an ongoing process of rehabilitation (or "habilitation" for those who have had no access to sound before).

This takes the form of two main streams:

Programming the device - so the user can hear sounds through it, and a Rehabilitation process - teaching the user to "make sense of" the sounds they're hearing.

Switch-on/Activation

This visit will take place 4 weeks following surgery. At this visit, the external speech processor is fitted and activated for the first time. This visit generally takes anywhere from 2-3 hours and it can be quite an emotional day for the patient and their family. While they will hear through the implant for the first time, the sound is likely to be very strange at first. It will take several weeks and months to get used to the new sound.

Programming

Programming can also be referred to as "tuning", or "mapping".

Subsequent Programming

Programming or Mapping of the implant will take place weekly for the first month, then at three months post-activation, then again at nine months post activation. Programming is when the audiologist works with the patient to determine the appropriate settings for the speech processor. A "Map" is created which tells the speech processor how to code the sound. Maps can change quite a bit over the first few weeks of implant use, so patients are seen frequently during this time. Maps are then monitored on a regular basis to ensure that the patient is receiving the highest quality sound that is possible for them.

Background

All implant users' hearing nerves will respond slightly differently to the electrical signals generated by the implant electrodes. Therefore "one size does not fit all". Consider two people with identical implants: for one person an electrical signal level of (e.g.) 300 units may represent a quiet sound. For the other person this same level could be very loud, or even uncomfortably loud. It all depends on their nerve's response to the signals.

Each implant user therefore needs a personalised set of information regarding their nerves' response. This information is termed a "Map" (or Programme) and is held in the speech processor's memory. The Map "tells" the processor that for this person, (e.g.) 300 units sounds quiet and (e.g.) 500 is loud. Therefore when the processor registers a quiet sound, a level of around 300 units should be sent to the nerve, and conversely, 500 for a loud sound. In this way the level (or loudness) of sounds the processor receives are mapped to the electrical levels that should be sent to the implant. However sound has another important characteristic: its frequency, or pitch. In cochlear implants this is represented primarily by using channels: Nearly all modern implants have a number of channels corresponding to the individual electrodes in the array. The speech processor splits the sound signal into these channels depending on the sound's pitch. Lower pitch sounds will be sent to electrodes deeper within the cochlea, and high pitch sounds to more shallowly placed electrodes. This mimics the way that the fully functioning inner ear responds, and helps to transmit information about the pitch of the sound to the implant user. Not only do the quiet / loud levels differ between people, they also differ to some degree between these channels. Therefore as above 300 units on one channel could be quiet but on another loud, even for the same person. So information on each channel is required.

So far levels have been described in terms of quiet and loud.

Each channel has three characteristics: Threshold, Comfortable Level, and Dynamic Range.

The Threshold is the lowest electrical level that causes a detectable sound sensation for the user. The lowest sound levels that the speech processor responds to will be mapped to electrical stimulation at this level, on this channel. The Comfortable Level is the highest electrical level that causes a sound sensation that is loud but still comfortable for the user (no-one wants to use a device causing uncomfortable stimulation). The highest sound levels that the speech processor responds to will be mapped to electrical stimulation at this level, on this channel.

The Dynamic Range is simply the difference between these two levels. The actual numbers or the size of the dynamic range are not too important. It is more important that the levels cause the right degree of loudness for the user. In this way sounds picked up by the processor will be mapped to the correct loudness levels giving the user the maximum information from the sound signal.

The speech processor samples incoming sounds many times a second, and sends corresponding electrical signals to the implant. Consider a sound that in this instant has a very high level in the low pitch area, a medium level at mid pitches, and a medium to high level at high pitches. In-between it's relatively quiet.

A further aspect of programming is which speech processing strategy is employed. This governs factors such as the rate at which information is sent to the channels and whether the channels are stimulated together or separately, as well as a number of other technical issues.

Determining these levels

Who does the task?

In most centres programming is carried out by audiologists: audiology technicians or audiological scientists. However other professionals with appropriate experience and training may be involved.

How are the levels found?

In most cases behavioural methods are used. This means that the CI user responds in some way to signals sent to their implant. Usually the speech processor will be interfaced to a computer running specialised software, and an automated check of the implant function (Telemetry) carried out. The user then wears their transmitting coil as normal. However they will not hear external sounds at this point, instead the computer generates electrical signals that are sent to the implant under the control of the audiologist.

Threshold: When programming adults, the audiologist presents the signals first at a level that the user should be able to easily detect so they become familiar with the task. The user responds whenever they hear a sound, perhaps by pressing a button, or simply by telling the audiologist they heard it. The audiologist adjusts the level until the lowest level at which the signal is detected is found. The process is repeated for the different channels.

Comfortable levels: With adults, the audiologist will increase the level and ask the user to indicate when it becomes loud but still comfortable. Alternatively the user can rate the sounds on a scale, i.e. quiet / medium / loud and comfortable / too loud, or similar.
In the very early days following implantation a cautious approach is taken and the audiologist may set comfortable levels at low electrical levels. This is to allow time to become accustomed to the new stimulation and avoid over-stimulating. This is especially important with younger children who need things to proceed at a pace suitable for them.

Time frame for programming

Usually quite a few appointments will be necessary in the first few months post-implantation, as a cautious approach is required. In addition some levels can change as the user adapts to the new stimulation - particularly the comfortable levels. As time goes on the appointments become less frequent. It is common though not always required for even well established users to attend yearly review appointments. Once all levels have stabilised and the audiologist is sure that the levels are correct the map is said to be optimal. There is no set time by which this has to be reached - again, it depends on the individual.

During the first few months of implant use a great deal of learning must take place. When initially switched-on, the implant may sound very strange and an individual may have quite a bit of difficulty understanding speech or identifying environmental sounds.

Habilitation sessions with a hearing therapist are offered for the first month of implant use and as needed after that to give the patient a chance to learn about their device and learn to use it effectively. Patients are encouraged to bring their significant other or a communication partner to these sessions as practice for home will be given. The patient and the hearing therapist may decide to continue the sessions longer than the first month if desired.

Habilitation Sessions

During the first few months of implant use a great deal of learning must take place. When initially switched-on, the implant may sound very strange and an individual may have quite a bit of difficulty understanding speech or identifying environmental sounds. Habilitation sessions with a hearing therapist are offered for the first month of implant use and as needed after that to give the patient a chance to learn about their device and learn to use it effectively. Patients are encouraged to bring their significant other or a communication partner to these sessions as practice for home will be given. The patient and the hearing therapist may decide to continue the sessions longer than the first month if desired.